THE QUICK FIX LOW SODIUM COOKBOOK

100 Recipes and Meal Plans for Easy, Delicious, and Heart Healthy Eating

Debra S. Elrod

TABLE OF CONTENTS

INTRODUCTION

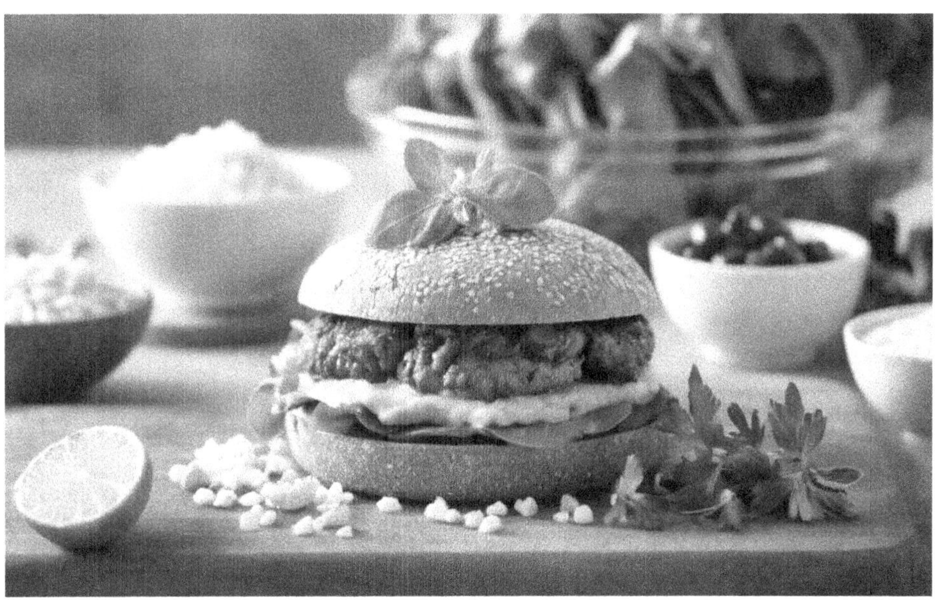

Welcome to The Quick Fix Low Sodium Cookbook

In a world where culinary pleasures often collide with health-conscious decisions, *The Quick Fix Low Sodium Cookbook* emerges as your culinary compass, guiding you towards a heart-healthy lifestyle without compromising on the joy of flavorful meals. As you embark on this journey, allow us to extend a warm welcome and introduce you to the enticing realm of low sodium cooking.

The Benefits of Embracing a Low Sodium Diet

Before we delve into the culinary treasures within these pages, let's take a moment to understand why embracing a low sodium diet is a choice worth making. This introduction is more than a mere prelude; it's a conversation about your well-being. A low sodium diet isn't just about cutting back on salt; it's a holistic approach to nurturing your heart and overall health. Discover how this dietary shift can have a profound impact on heart health, going beyond just lowering blood pressure.

Chapter 1: Understanding the Advantages

Our first chapter is a journey into the advantages of adopting a low sodium diet. We unravel the intricate connections between sodium intake and heart health. By exploring the impact on blood pressure and beyond, we lay the foundation for making informed decisions about what goes on your plate. Knowledge is a powerful tool, and in this chapter, you'll gain insights that empower you to take control of your health.

Chapter 2: Recipes and Meal Plans

The heart of the cookbook unfolds in this expansive chapter, where we present a curated collection of 100 recipes and meal plans designed to tantalize your taste buds and nourish your body. From the first light of morning through the savory midday and into the evening repast, explore the diversity of flavors and culinary experiences that await you.

- **Breakfast**: Rise and shine with a variety of morning delights that go beyond the typical low sodium fare. From energizing smoothies to hearty breakfast bowls, discover how to start your day with flavor and health in mind.

- **Lunch**: Our lunchtime inspirations offer 35 options that strike the perfect balance between delicious and heart-healthy. Whether you prefer salads, sandwiches, or warm bowls, there's something here to satisfy every palate.

- **Dinner**: As the day winds down, savor 40 dinner creations that make low sodium dining a culinary adventure. From quick weeknight dinners to more elaborate weekend feasts, each recipe is crafted with your health and enjoyment in mind.

- **A 7-Day Low Sodium Meal Plan**: Simplify your week with our carefully crafted meal plan, ensuring a variety of flavors and nutrients while adhering to your heart-healthy goals. Follow along for a seamless and delicious week of wholesome eating.

Chapter 3: Simple Strategies To Cut Your Sodium Intake

Reducing sodium doesn't mean compromising on taste. In this chapter, we provide you with practical strategies to cut back on sodium in your everyday cooking. From smart ingredient swaps to ingenious flavor enhancers that go beyond salt, you'll discover that a low sodium lifestyle can be both health-conscious and incredibly flavorful.

Chapter 4: Dispelling Myths Around Salt Consumption

Let's debunk some common myths surrounding salt consumption. It's time to separate fact from fiction and gain clarity on what really matters when it comes to sodium in our diets. Understanding these myths is key to making informed choices that align with your health goals.

Let Get Started

The Benefits of Embracing a Low Sodium Diet

Understanding the Everyday Impact

Have you ever paused to reflect on the subtle dance of flavors that grace your plate? Every bite tells a story, and your journey begins with a simple shift – a commitment to a low sodium diet. Beyond the immediate allure of delectable recipes lies a tapestry of health benefits that touch the very core of your well-being.

Consider your heart, that resilient organ orchestrating the rhythm of your life. Embracing a low sodium diet is like offering it a gentle, loving symphony. As we navigate the intricacies of this culinary expedition, let's uncover the harmonious notes that echo through every beat of your heart.

Heart Health: More Than a Metaphor

Our hearts aren't just symbols of love; they are the epicenters of our vitality. Picture your heart as a dedicated worker, tirelessly pumping life through your veins. Now, imagine the burdens it bears when faced with an excess of sodium, that often unnoticed culprit lurking in many of our daily meals.

As we unravel the benefits of a low sodium diet, we find an immediate ally in maintaining heart health. The impact on blood pressure becomes a gentle ebb rather than a tumultuous surge. It's a whispered promise that your heart will thank you for, a pledge to support its tireless efforts with meals that nurture rather than strain.

Beyond the Pulse: Holistic Health Improvements

Yet, the advantages extend beyond the rhythmic beats of your heart. Embracing a low sodium diet becomes a holistic gesture, an act of self-love that reverberates through various facets of your well-being. Picture a cascade of positive effects – lowered risk of cardiovascular diseases, improved kidney function, and enhanced overall vitality.

In this journey, your body becomes a cherished companion, responding to the nourishment of flavors that don't compromise health for taste. It's about recognizing that every choice, every forkful, is an investment in the longevity and vibrancy of your life.

Personal Stories: A Tapestry of Wellness

The beauty of embracing a low sodium diet lies not just in the scientific insights but in the narratives of everyday individuals. It's in the stories of those who found renewed energy, better sleep, and a zest for life simply by altering their approach to food.

Take Jane, a spirited mother of two, who discovered that by embracing a low sodium lifestyle, she not only safeguarded her heart health but also became a role model for her children. Or consider Mike, a busy professional, who found that the simple act of reducing sodium in his meals translated to increased focus and productivity.

These are not distant tales but the echoes of lives transformed, illustrating that the benefits of a low sodium diet are not confined to a select few. They are an inclusive celebration of improved well-being, a testament to the universal impact of mindful and heart-conscious eating.

The Flavorful Equation: A Symphony of Tastes

Now, you might wonder, does adopting a low sodium diet mean bidding farewell to the pleasures of taste? Absolutely not! In fact, it's an invitation to a richer, more nuanced culinary experience. It's about embracing the myriad flavors that dance on your palate without the overpowering presence of excess salt.

In the pages of *The Quick Fix Low Sodium Cookbook*, you'll encounter recipes that tantalize your taste buds, proving that health and flavor need not be mutually exclusive. Imagine savoring a perfectly seasoned dish, where each ingredient shines in its natural brilliance. It's about rediscovering the joy of eating, one delicious bite at a time.

The Ripple Effect: A Journey Beyond the Plate

As you embark on this journey of low sodium living, it's essential to acknowledge the ripple effect it creates. The choices we make in our kitchens echo not only in our personal health but in the broader canvas of societal well-being. By choosing a low sodium path, you contribute to a collective shift towards healthier living, inspiring others to embark on their wellness odyssey.

Consider the impact on future generations as you pass down not just recipes but a legacy of mindful eating. It's a legacy that speaks volumes about the connection between flavor, health, and the joy of savoring life's simple, yet profound, pleasures.

Closing Thoughts: Your Personal Invitation

So here you are, at the threshold of a culinary adventure that transcends the ordinary. Embracing a low sodium diet is not just a choice; it's an affirmation of your commitment to a life well-lived. It's about savoring the journey as much as the flavors on your plate.

As you flip through the pages of *The Quick Fix Low Sodium Cookbook*, may you feel a sense of empowerment, a personal invitation to prioritize your health without sacrificing the pleasure of eating. Your well-being is not just a goal; it's a delicious and heartwarming journey, and we are thrilled to be part of it. Cheers to the joy of mindful, heart-healthy living, and to the vibrant chapters that unfold as you embrace the benefits of a low sodium diet!

SELF-REFLECTION QUESTIONS

- What motivated you to explore the concept of a low sodium diet, and how do you envision its impact on your personal health journey?

- As you absorb the information about the benefits of embracing a low sodium diet, what aspects resonate with your current health goals and lifestyle choices?

UNDERSTANDING THE ADVANTAGES

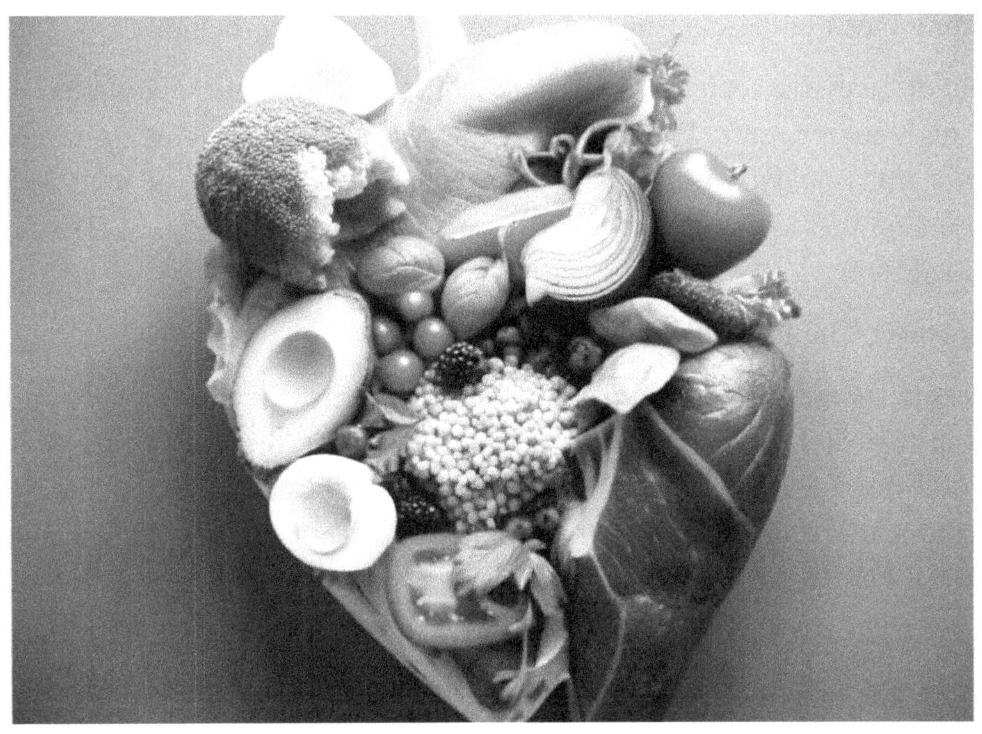

The Impact of Low Sodium Diet on Heart Health, A Deep Dive into Cardiovascular Well-being

In the symphony of our bodily functions, the heart plays the lead role, orchestrating the rhythm of life. It's not just an organ; it's a pulsating metaphor for vitality and health. As we embark on a journey to understand the profound impact of a low sodium diet on heart health, let's explore the intricacies of this relationship and uncover the symphony that unfolds with every beat.

The Heart as a Conductor

Imagine your heart as a conductor, guiding a complex orchestra of blood vessels, each carrying the life force that sustains us. Like a maestro shaping a symphony, the heart orchestrates the circulation of blood, ensuring that every cell receives the nutrients and oxygen it needs. However, this intricate dance can be disrupted by the silent intruder that is sodium.

Sodium: The Stealthy Intruder

Sodium, a seemingly innocuous element, holds the potential to disrupt the harmonious composition of our cardiovascular symphony. It's a common ingredient in our diets, often hiding in plain sight. From processed foods to restaurant meals, sodium sneaks into our plates, adding flavor but also posing a threat to our heart's well-being.

The impact of excessive sodium intake on heart health is primarily manifested through its influence on blood pressure. Picture your blood vessels as the highways through which blood flows, carrying vital nutrients and oxygen to every corner of your body. When there's an excess of sodium, these blood vessels can constrict, creating resistance to the flow of blood.

Blood Pressure: The Pressure Points

Blood pressure is the force exerted by the blood against the walls of the arteries. It's measured in two values: systolic pressure (the force when the heart beats) and diastolic pressure (the force when the heart is at rest between beats). When sodium levels are elevated, the body retains more water to dilute the excess sodium. This increased fluid volume puts a strain on the walls of the arteries, leading to an elevation in blood pressure.

Consistently high blood pressure can have far-reaching consequences for heart health. It places undue stress on the heart, compelling it to work harder to pump blood. Over time, this extra workload can lead to the thickening of the heart muscle, a condition known as left ventricular hypertrophy. Left untreated, it can pave the way for more severe cardiovascular issues, including heart failure.

Low Sodium Diet as a Heart-Health Hero

Now, let's shift our focus to the hero of our narrative—the low sodium diet. Embracing a diet low in sodium is like extending a caring hand to your heart, alleviating the burdens placed upon it. By reducing sodium intake, we create an environment where blood vessels can relax, allowing blood to flow more freely.

Imagine your arteries as waterways, unobstructed and flowing smoothly, nourishing every cell in their path. A low sodium diet contributes to the maintenance of healthy blood pressure levels, relieving the heart of unnecessary strain. It's a compassionate choice that empowers the heart to beat with ease, sustaining the symphony of life without the discordant notes of hypertension.

The Unseen Culprits: Processed and Packaged Foods

To truly understand the impact of a low sodium diet, we must confront the culprits that often contribute to excessive sodium consumption. Processed and packaged foods, convenient though they may be, are often laden with hidden sodium. From canned soups to ready-to-eat meals, these products can significantly contribute to daily sodium intake without the diner even realizing it.

Navigating the modern food landscape requires a discerning eye. Reading labels becomes an essential skill, as sodium content is often camouflaged under various names. A low sodium diet involves a conscious effort to choose fresh, whole foods over their processed counterparts. It's a return to the basics of cooking and a rediscovery of the inherent flavors of natural ingredients.

Elevating Flavor, Lowering Sodium

One common misconception about low sodium diets is that they equate to bland and tasteless meals. However, this couldn't be further from the truth. The journey toward a heart-healthy, low sodium lifestyle invites us to explore a vibrant palette of herbs, spices, and creative flavor enhancers that elevate our culinary experiences.

Think of it as a culinary adventure where you become the master chef of your heart-healthy kitchen. Swap out the salt shaker for a spectrum of aromatic spices—rosemary, thyme, cumin, and paprika—to infuse your dishes with depth and character. Embracing a low sodium diet is not about sacrificing flavor; it's about enhancing it in a way that is mindful of your heart's well-being.

Lowering Blood Pressure and Beyond

The Silent Struggle of High Blood Pressure

High blood pressure, or hypertension, is often referred to as the *"silent killer"* for good reason. It can quietly wreak havoc on our cardiovascular system, often without presenting noticeable symptoms. The heart, in its ceaseless effort to pump blood throughout the body, encounters increased resistance when blood vessels narrow due to excessive sodium levels.

Imagine this resistance as a persistent force against the walls of your arteries. Over time, it can lead to the wear and tear of these vessels, setting the stage for potential cardiovascular complications. Lowering blood pressure is not just a numerical goal; it's a profound strategy to reduce the strain on the heart and mitigate the risk of more severe health issues.

The Ripple Effect of Lower Blood Pressure

Embracing a low sodium diet is like applying a soothing balm to the cardiovascular system. As blood pressure stabilizes, a cascade of positive effects begins to unfold, influencing various aspects of our health.

1. Cardiovascular Resilience: The Heart's Symphony

The heart, our tireless conductor, orchestrates the symphony of our circulatory system. With lower blood pressure, the heart encounters less resistance, allowing it to beat more efficiently. This enhanced efficiency contributes to the overall cardiovascular resilience, reducing the strain on the heart muscle and promoting long-term heart health.

2. Preservation of Arterial Health: The Vascular Canvas

Picture your arteries as a delicate canvas, with blood flowing gracefully through them. High blood pressure is akin to subjecting this canvas to constant turbulence. Lowering blood pressure through a low sodium diet helps preserve the integrity of your arteries, maintaining their flexibility and reducing the risk of arterial damage.

3. Mitigating the Risk of Stroke: A Protective Shield

High blood pressure is a significant risk factor for strokes, often referred to as "brain attacks." The delicately balanced circulation that nourishes our brains becomes vulnerable when blood pressure is consistently elevated. Adopting a low sodium lifestyle acts as a protective shield, mitigating the risk of strokes and safeguarding the intricate network of vessels that support cognitive health.

Expanding the Canvas: Beyond Blood Pressure

While the reduction of blood pressure is a critical milestone, the benefits of a low sodium diet extend beyond this focal point. Let's explore the broader canvas of advantages that await those who choose the path of low sodium living.

1. Kidney Health: Filtering with Precision

Our kidneys, the unsung heroes of filtration, play a pivotal role in maintaining the body's fluid and electrolyte balance. The delicate dance between sodium and potassium is intricately regulated by these vital organs. Excessive sodium intake can burden the kidneys, potentially leading to conditions such as kidney stones or impaired function. A low sodium diet eases this burden, allowing the kidneys to filter with precision and promoting optimal renal health.

2. Fluid Balance: Alleviating Bloating and Discomfort

Have you ever experienced that post-meal bloating, the discomfort that lingers after indulging in a sodium-rich feast? A low sodium diet is your ticket to alleviating this common woe. By promoting fluid balance, it reduces water retention, offering a sense of lightness and ease in your daily life. It's a simple yet impactful way to enhance your overall comfort and well-being.

3. Weight Management: A Supportive Ally

Weight management is a multifaceted journey, and a low sodium diet can be a supportive ally in this endeavor. Excessive sodium consumption can contribute to water weight gain, creating a temporary but noticeable increase on the scale. By adopting a low sodium lifestyle, you contribute to a more accurate reflection of your body's true composition, facilitating a holistic approach to weight management.

4. Preservation of Endothelial Function: Nurturing the Inner Lining

The endothelium, the inner lining of blood vessels, plays a crucial role in maintaining vascular health. High sodium levels can impair endothelial function, potentially leading to inflammation and oxidative stress. A low sodium diet nurtures the endothelium, preserving its integrity and contributing to the overall health of your blood vessels.

5. Joint Health: Easing Discomfort

Sodium can contribute to inflammation in the body, affecting not only blood vessels but also joints. Individuals with conditions such as arthritis may find relief in a low sodium diet, as it can help reduce inflammation and alleviate joint discomfort. It's a holistic approach to well-being that extends beyond cardiovascular health.

LOW SODIUM BREAKFAST RECIPES

Oatmeal with Fresh Berries:

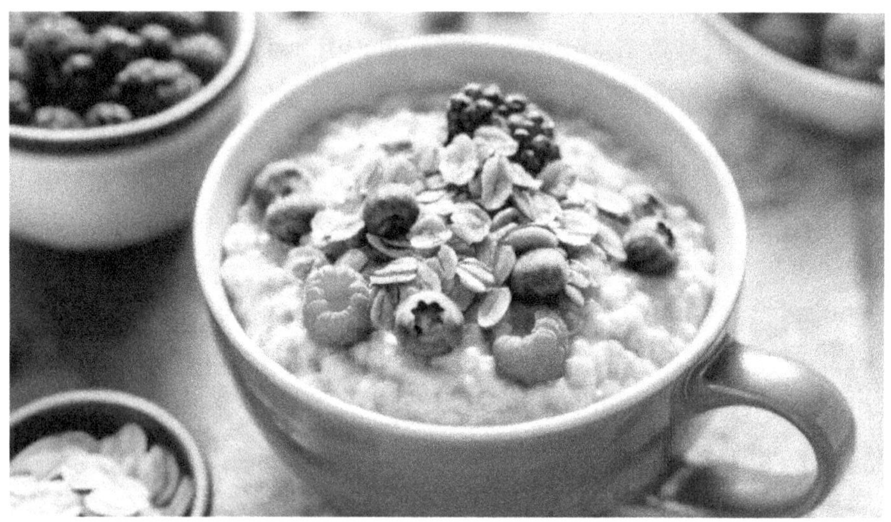

Ingredients: Rolled oats, water or low sodium milk, fresh berries.

Preparation: Cook oats with water or milk, top with fresh berries.

Greek Yogurt Parfait:

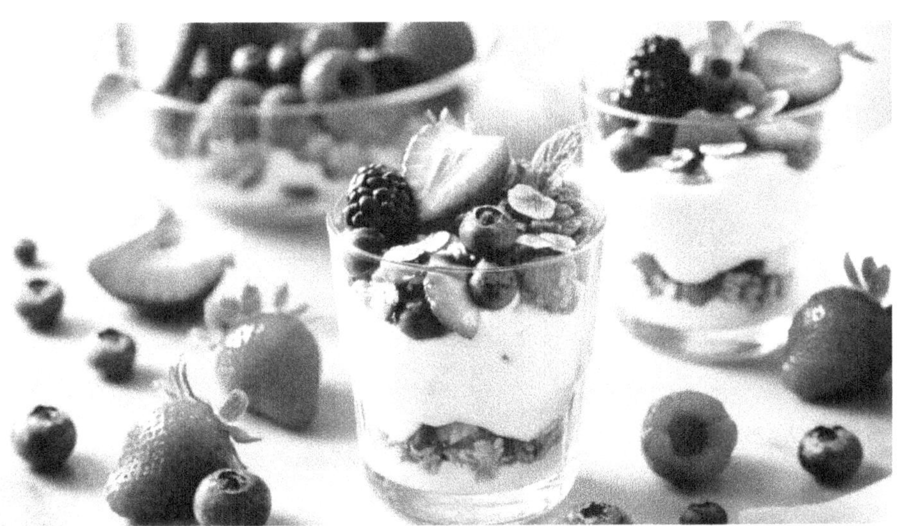

Ingredients: Greek yogurt, granola (low sodium), mixed fruit.

Preparation: Layer Greek yogurt with low sodium granola and mixed fruit.

Avocado Toast:

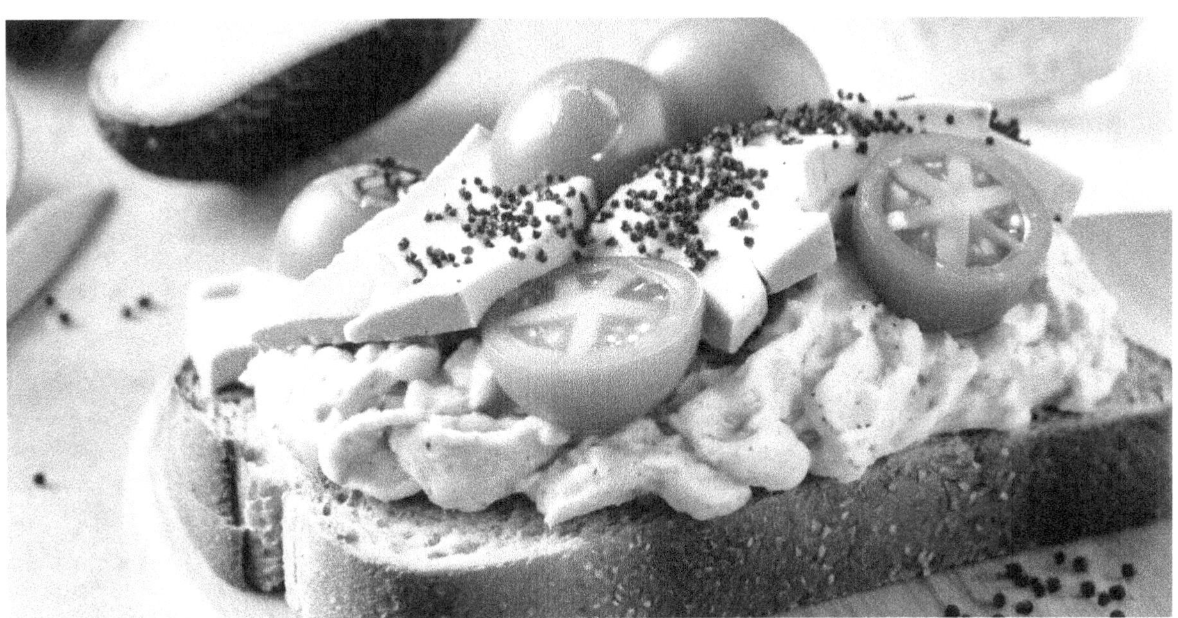

Ingredients: Whole-grain bread, avocado, cherry tomatoes, black pepper.

Preparation: Toast bread, spread mashed avocado, top with sliced tomatoes, and sprinkle with black pepper.

Egg White Omelette:

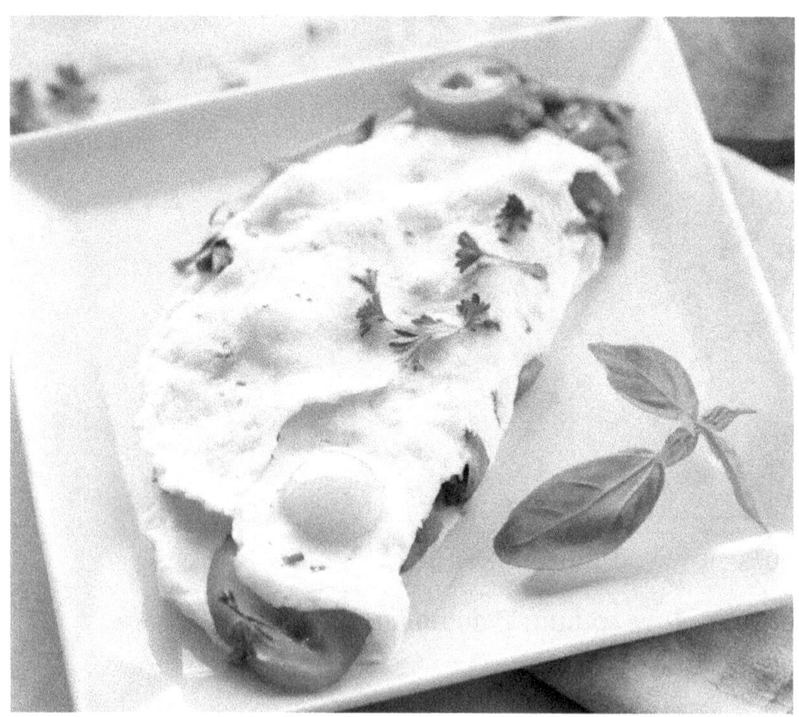

Ingredients: Egg whites, spinach, tomatoes, feta cheese.

Preparation: Whisk egg whites, pour into a pan with spinach, tomatoes, and feta; fold into an omelette.

Smoothie Bowl:

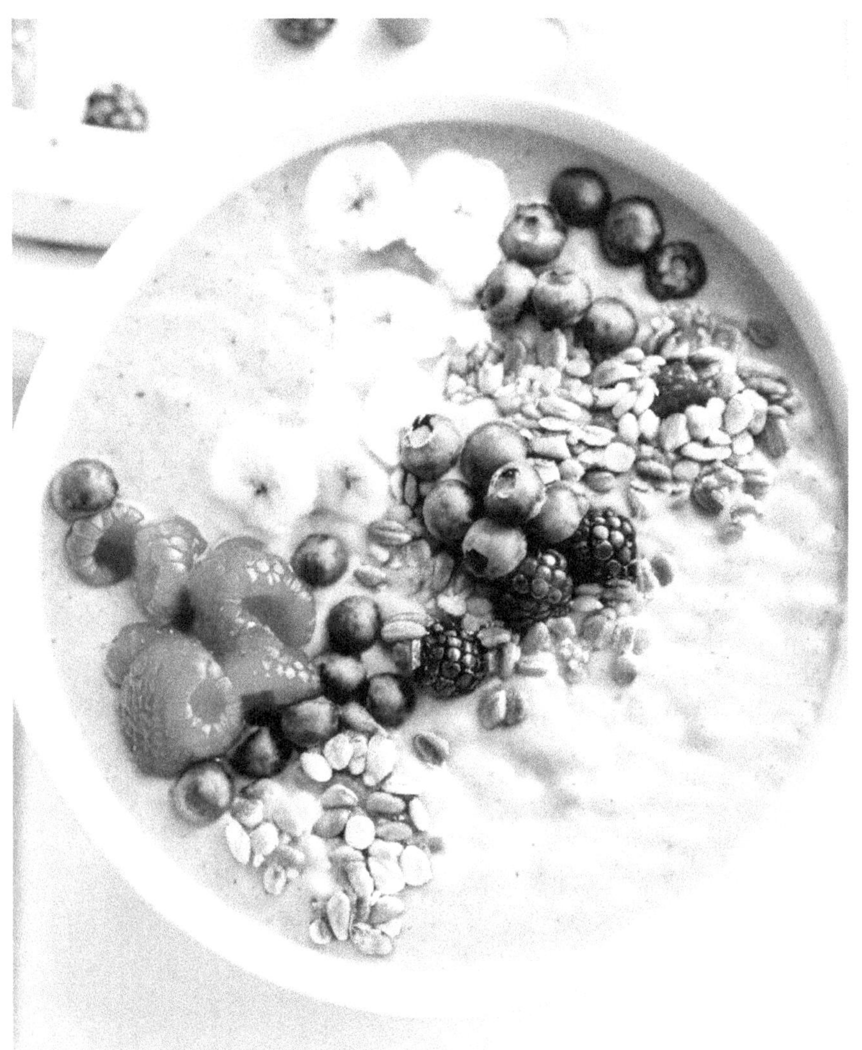

Ingredients: Frozen mixed berries, banana, low sodium yogurt.

Preparation: Blend berries, banana, and yogurt; top with nuts and seeds.

Quinoa Breakfast Bowl:

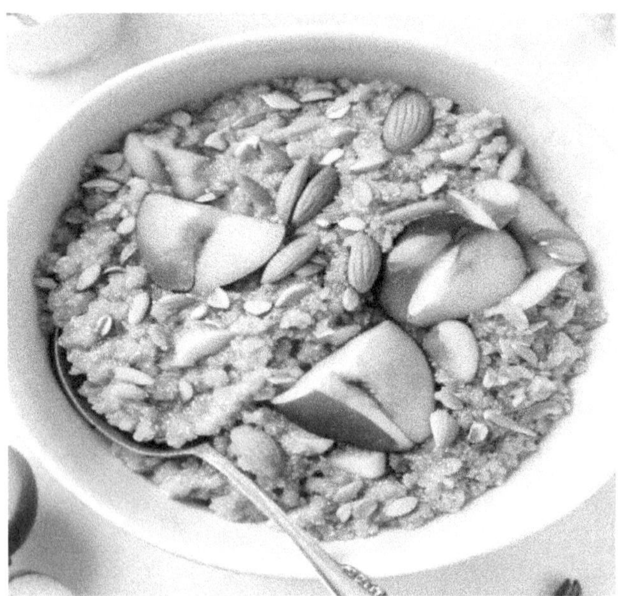

Ingredients: Quinoa, almond milk, sliced peaches, cinnamon.

Preparation: Cook quinoa in almond milk, top with sliced peaches and a sprinkle of cinnamon.

Chia Seed Pudding:

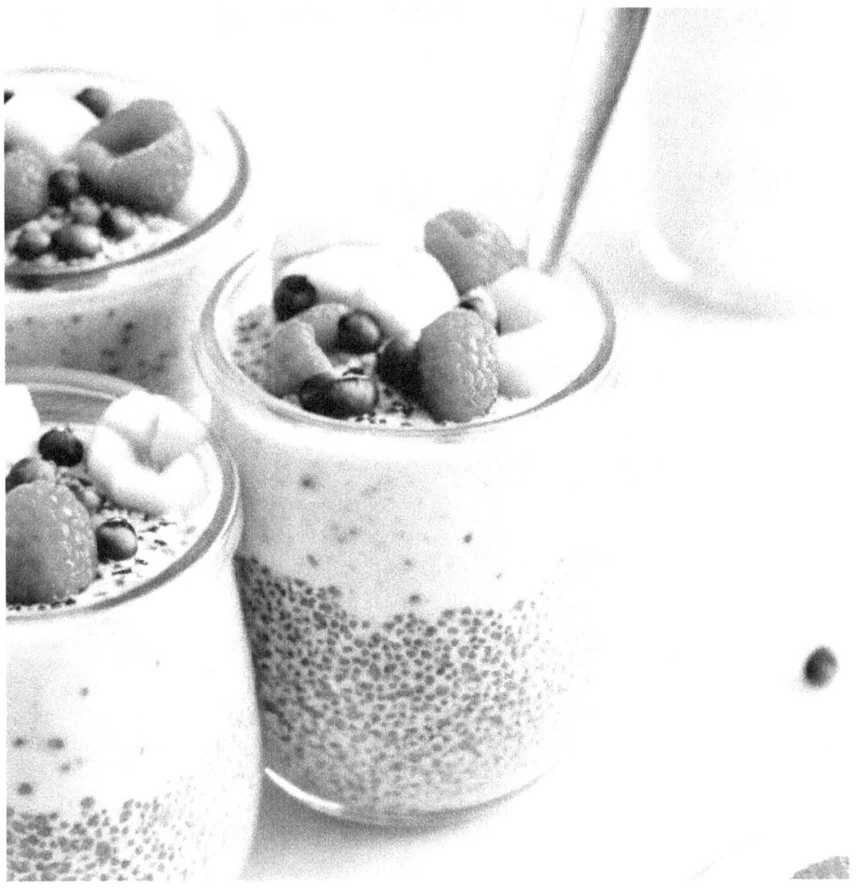

Ingredients: Chia seeds, coconut milk, sliced mango.

Preparation: Mix chia seeds with coconut milk, refrigerate overnight, and top with sliced mango.

Whole Grain Pancakes:

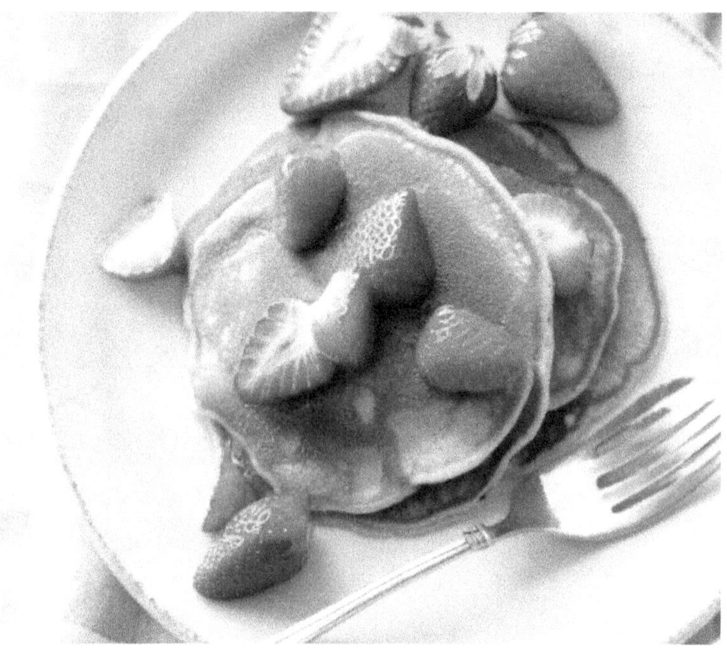

Ingredients: Whole grain pancake mix, low sodium syrup, fresh strawberries.

Preparation: Prepare pancakes, top with fresh strawberries and a drizzle of low sodium syrup.

Breakfast Burrito:

Ingredients: Whole wheat tortilla, scrambled eggs, black beans, salsa.

Preparation: Fill a tortilla with scrambled eggs, black beans, and salsa.

Cottage Cheese with Pineapple:

Ingredients: Low sodium cottage cheese, fresh pineapple.

Preparation: Mix cottage cheese with fresh pineapple chunks.

Sweet Potato Hash:

Ingredients: Sweet potatoes, bell peppers, onions, olive oil.

Preparation: Sauté diced sweet potatoes, bell peppers, and onions in olive oil.

Homemade Muesli:

Ingredients: Rolled oats, nuts, seeds, dried fruit.

Preparation: Mix oats, nuts, seeds, and dried fruit; serve with low sodium milk.

Spinach and Feta Frittata:

Ingredients: Eggs, spinach, feta cheese.

Preparation: Whisk eggs, mix with spinach and feta; bake until set.

Peanut Butter Banana Toast:

Ingredients: Whole-grain bread, peanut butter, banana slices.

Preparation: Toast bread, spread with peanut butter, and top with banana slices.

Ricotta Berry Toast:

Ingredients: Whole-grain bread, ricotta cheese, mixed berries.

Preparation: Toast bread, spread with ricotta, and top with mixed berries.

Chickpea and Veggie Scramble:

Ingredients: Chickpeas, bell peppers, tomatoes, cumin.

Preparation: Sauté chickpeas with bell peppers and tomatoes, season with cumin.

Baked Apple Oatmeal:

Ingredients: Rolled oats, apples, cinnamon, almond milk.

Preparation: Mix oats with diced apples, cinnamon, and almond milk; bake until golden.

Blueberry Banana Protein Smoothie:

Ingredients: Blueberries, banana, protein powder, almond milk.

Preparation: Blend blueberries, banana, protein powder, and almond milk.

Yogurt and Berry Parfait:

Ingredients: Low sodium yogurt, strawberries, blueberries.

Preparation: Layer yogurt with sliced strawberries and blueberries.

Cranberry Almond Quinoa Bowl:

Ingredients: Quinoa, cranberries, almonds, honey.

Preparation: Mix cooked quinoa with cranberries and almonds; drizzle with honey.

Cherry Almond Smoothie:

Ingredients: Cherries, almond butter, low sodium yogurt.

Preparation: Blend cherries, almond butter, and yogurt until smooth.

Egg and Veggie Wrap:

Ingredients: Whole wheat wrap, scrambled eggs, bell peppers, salsa.

Preparation: Fill a wrap with scrambled eggs, bell peppers, and salsa.

Mango Coconut Chia Pudding:

Ingredients: Chia seeds, coconut milk, diced mango.

Preparation: Mix chia seeds with coconut milk, refrigerate, and top with diced mango.

Peach and Almond Overnight Oats:

Ingredients: Rolled oats, almond milk, sliced peaches.

Preparation: Combine oats with almond milk and peaches; refrigerate overnight.

Caprese Avocado Toast:

Ingredients: Whole-grain bread, avocado, cherry tomatoes, mozzarella.

Preparation: Toast bread, spread with mashed avocado, top with tomatoes and mozzarella.

Strawberry Banana Protein Pancakes:

Ingredients: Whole grain pancake mix, strawberries, banana, protein powder.

Preparation: Prepare pancakes with protein powder; top with sliced strawberries and banana.

Pumpkin Spice Chia Pudding:

Ingredients: Chia seeds, pumpkin puree, almond milk, cinnamon.

Preparation: Mix chia seeds with pumpkin puree, almond milk, and cinnamon; refrigerate.

Mango Tango Smoothie Bowl:

Ingredients: Mango, low sodium yogurt, granola.

Preparation: Blend mango and yogurt; pour into a bowl and top with granola.

Cinnamon Raisin Overnight Oats:

Ingredients: Rolled oats, almond milk, cinnamon, raisins.

Preparation: Mix oats with almond milk, cinnamon, and raisins; refrigerate overnight.

Almond Butter and Banana Wrap:

Ingredients: Whole wheat wrap, almond butter, banana.

Preparation: Spread almond butter on a wrap, add sliced banana, and roll it up.

LOW-SODIUM LUNCH RECIPES

Grilled Chicken Salad:

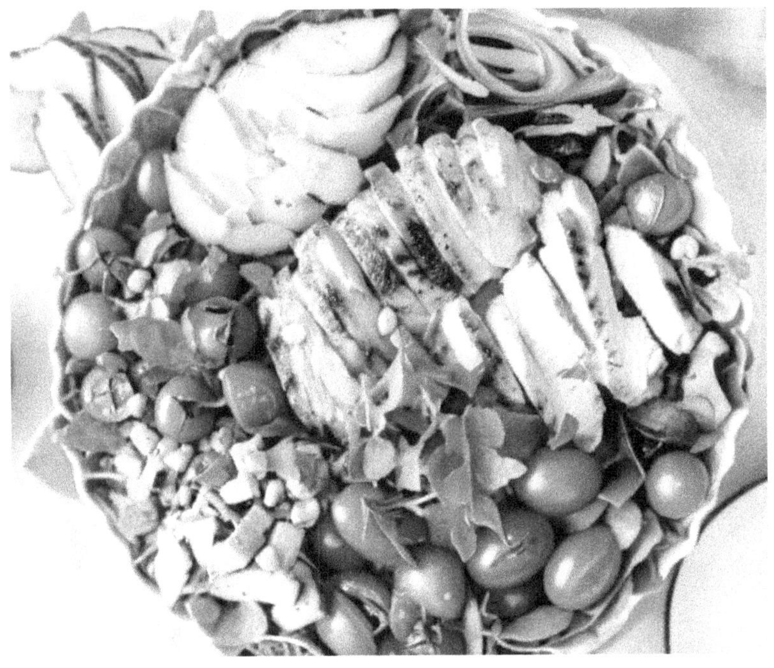

Ingredients: Grilled chicken breast, mixed greens, cherry tomatoes, cucumber.

Preparation: Toss grilled chicken with mixed greens, cherry tomatoes, and sliced cucumber.

Quinoa and Black Bean Bowl:

Ingredients: Quinoa, black beans, corn, bell peppers.

Preparation: Mix cooked quinoa with black beans, corn, and diced bell peppers.

Salmon and Asparagus Foil Pack:

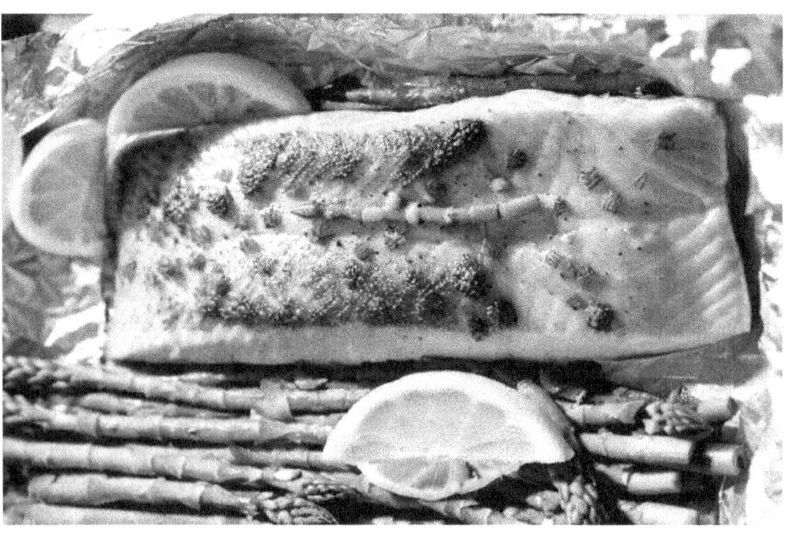

Ingredients: Salmon fillet, asparagus, lemon.

Preparation: Place salmon and asparagus in a foil pack, squeeze lemon over, and bake.

Vegetarian Wrap:

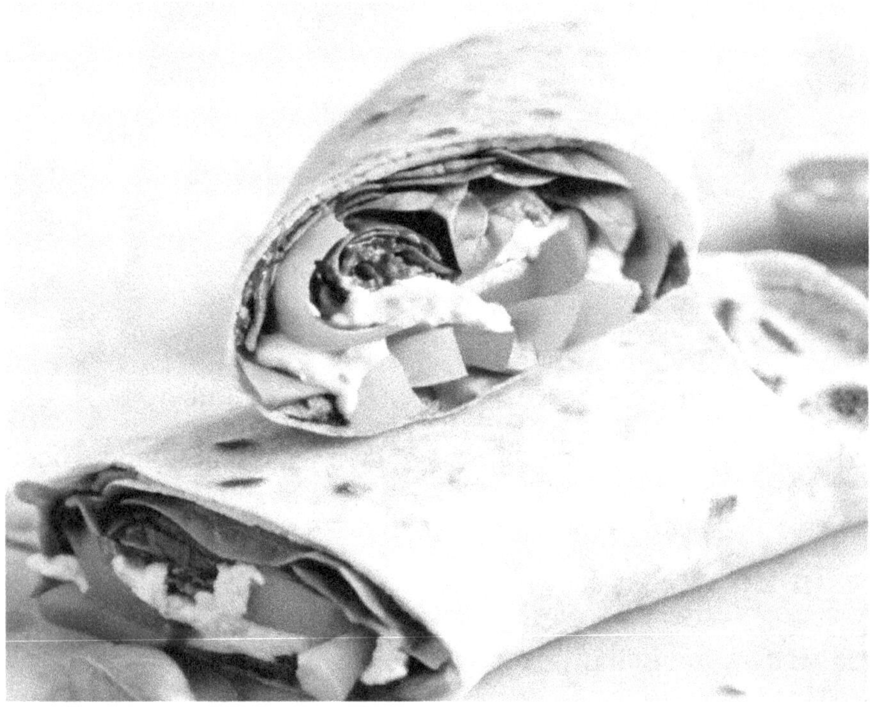

Ingredients: Whole wheat wrap, hummus, spinach, bell peppers.

Preparation: Spread hummus on a wrap, add spinach and sliced bell peppers, then roll it up.

Mediterranean Chickpea Salad:

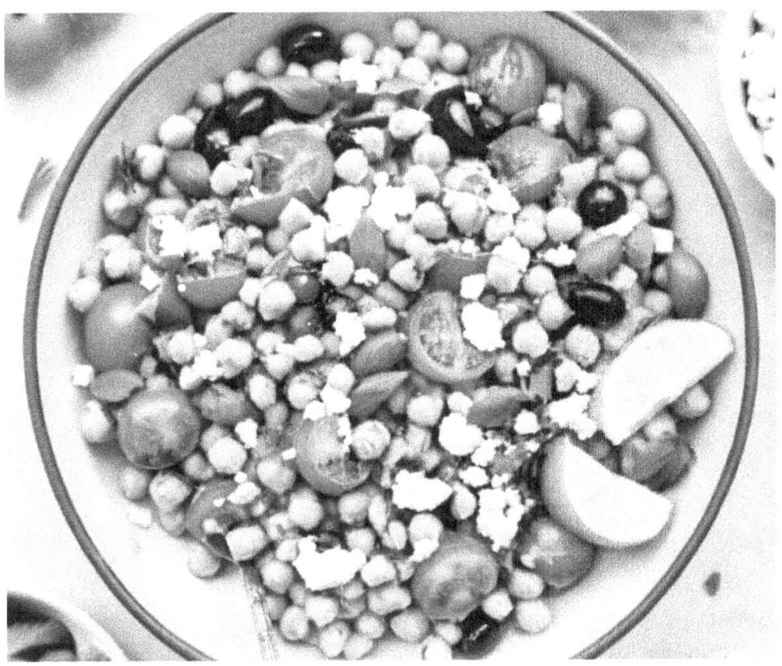

Ingredients: Chickpeas, cherry tomatoes, feta cheese, olives.

Preparation: Combine chickpeas with halved cherry tomatoes, feta cheese, and olives.

Turkey and Avocado Lettuce Wraps:

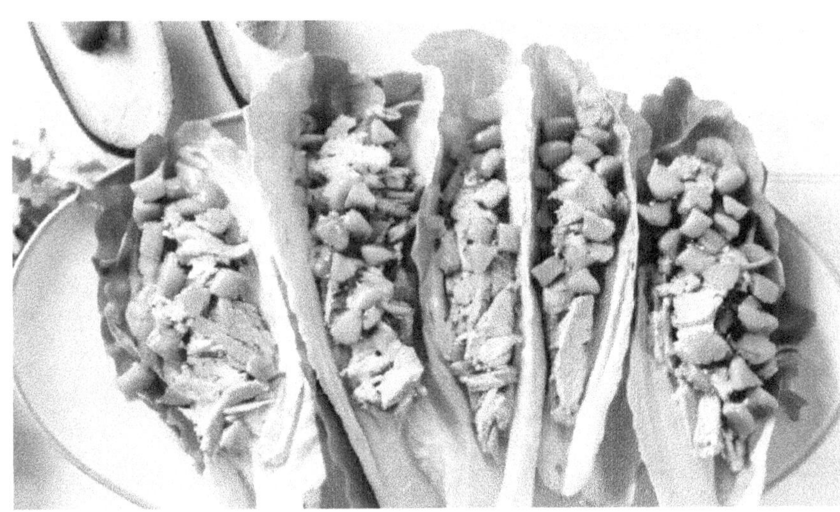

Ingredients: Turkey slices, lettuce leaves, avocado.

Preparation: Wrap turkey slices and sliced avocado in lettuce leaves.

Brown Rice and Vegetable Stir-Fry:

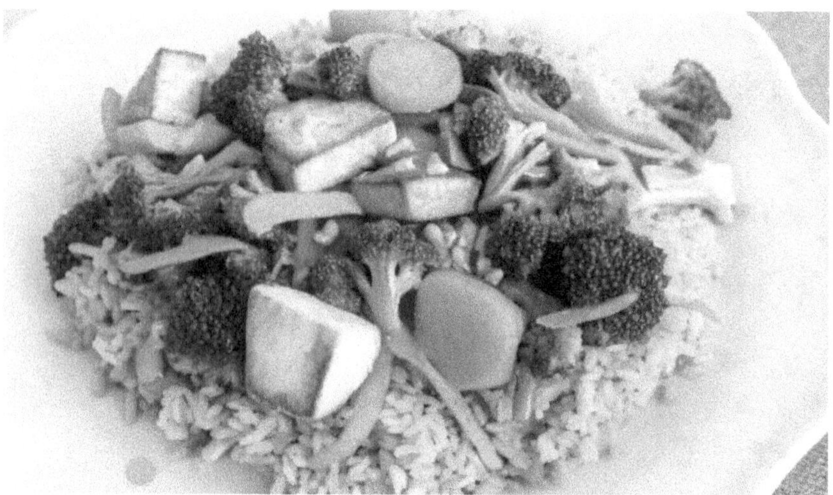

Ingredients: Brown rice, broccoli, carrots, tofu.

Preparation: Stir-fry cooked brown rice with broccoli, carrots, and tofu.

Cauliflower and Chickpea Curry:

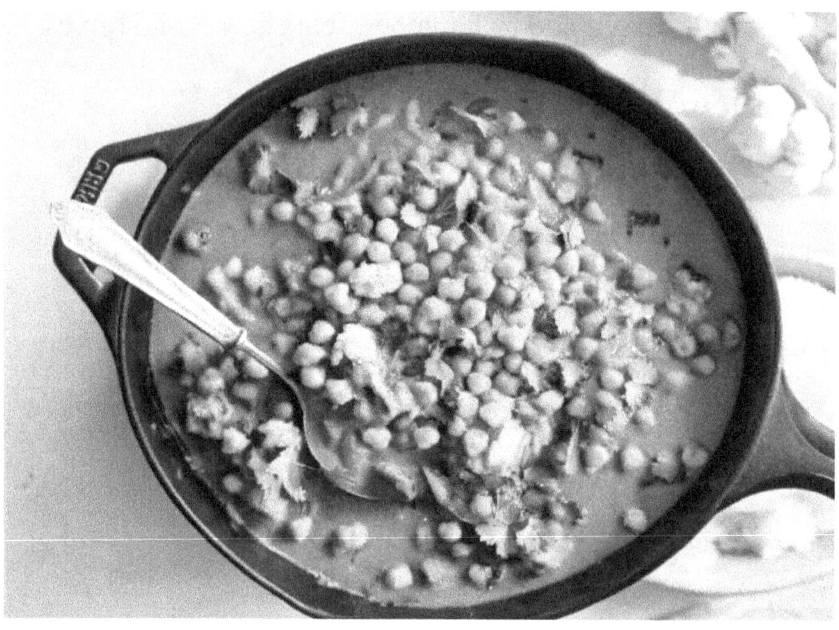

Ingredients: Cauliflower, chickpeas, coconut milk, curry spices.

Preparation: Cook cauliflower and chickpeas in coconut milk with curry spices.

Caprese Quinoa Salad:

Ingredients: Quinoa, cherry tomatoes, mozzarella, basil.

Preparation: Combine cooked quinoa with halved cherry tomatoes, mozzarella, and basil.

Egg Salad Lettuce Wraps:

Ingredients: Hard-boiled eggs, lettuce leaves, Greek yogurt.

Preparation: Mix chopped hard-boiled eggs with Greek yogurt, then wrap in lettuce leaves.

Shrimp and Zucchini Noodles:

Ingredients: Shrimp, zucchini, garlic, olive oil.

Preparation: Sauté shrimp and zucchini noodles with garlic in olive oil.

Sweet Potato and Lentil Stew:

Ingredients: Sweet potatoes, lentils, vegetable broth, cumin.

Preparation: Cook sweet potatoes and lentils in vegetable broth with cumin.

Tuna and White Bean Salad:

Ingredients: Canned tuna, white beans, red onion, parsley.

Preparation: Mix canned tuna with white beans, diced red onion, and chopped parsley.

Tomato and Basil Whole Wheat Pasta:

Ingredients: Whole wheat pasta, cherry tomatoes, fresh basil.

Preparation: Toss cooked whole wheat pasta with halved cherry tomatoes and fresh basil.

Stuffed Bell Peppers with Ground Turkey:

Ingredients: Bell peppers, ground turkey, brown rice, tomato sauce.

Preparation: Fill bell peppers with a mixture of cooked ground turkey, brown rice, and tomato sauce.

Cucumber and Tofu Salad:

Ingredients: Cucumber, tofu, sesame seeds, soy sauce.

Preparation: Combine sliced cucumber and tofu, sprinkle with sesame seeds, and drizzle with soy sauce.

Greek Chicken Pita Pocket:

Ingredients: Grilled chicken, whole wheat pita, Greek yogurt, cucumber.

Preparation: Fill a whole wheat pita with grilled chicken, Greek yogurt, and sliced cucumber.

Vegetable and Bean Quesadilla:

Ingredients: Whole wheat tortilla, black beans, bell peppers, cheese.

Preparation: Layer black beans, sliced bell peppers, and cheese between whole wheat tortillas, then cook until cheese melts.

Lemon Garlic Shrimp Salad:

Ingredients: Shrimp, mixed greens, lemon, garlic.

Preparation: Sauté shrimp with minced garlic, serve over mixed greens, and squeeze lemon on top.

Chickpea and Spinach Wrap:

Ingredients: Whole wheat wrap, chickpeas, spinach, tahini.

Preparation: Fill a wrap with chickpeas, spinach, and a drizzle of tahini.

Cabbage and Carrot Slaw with Turkey:

Ingredients: Shredded cabbage, shredded carrots, ground turkey.

Preparation: Sauté ground turkey, serve over a slaw of shredded cabbage and carrots.

Stuffed Portobello Mushrooms:

Ingredients: Portobello mushrooms, quinoa, feta cheese, spinach.

Preparation: Fill portobello mushrooms with a mixture of cooked quinoa, feta cheese, and sautéed spinach.

Vegetarian Lentil Soup:

Ingredients: Lentils, carrots, celery, vegetable broth.

Preparation: Cook lentils with diced carrots and celery in vegetable broth.

Tofu and Vegetable Skewers:

Ingredients: Tofu, bell peppers, cherry tomatoes, balsamic glaze.

Preparation: Thread tofu, bell peppers, and cherry tomatoes onto skewers, grill, and drizzle with balsamic glaze.

Broccoli and Brown Rice Casserole:

Ingredients: Brown rice, broccoli, low sodium cheese.

Preparation: Mix cooked brown rice and steamed broccoli, top with low sodium cheese, and bake until melted.

Cilantro Lime Chicken Salad:

Ingredients: Grilled chicken, mixed greens, cilantro, lime.

Preparation: Toss grilled chicken with mixed greens, chopped cilantro, and a squeeze of lime.

Veggie and Hummus Wrap:

Ingredients: Whole wheat wrap, hummus, bell peppers, cucumber.

Preparation: Spread hummus on a wrap, add sliced bell peppers and cucumber, and roll it up.

Sesame Ginger Tofu Stir-Fry:

Ingredients: Tofu, broccoli, snow peas, sesame ginger sauce.

Preparation: Stir-fry tofu, broccoli, and snow peas with sesame ginger sauce.

Couscous and Chickpea Salad:

Ingredients: Couscous, chickpeas, cherry tomatoes, parsley.

Preparation: Combine cooked couscous with chickpeas, halved cherry tomatoes, and chopped parsley.

Spaghetti Squash with Marinara Sauce:

Ingredients: Spaghetti squash, marinara sauce, basil.

Preparation: Roast spaghetti squash, shred into strands, and top with marinara sauce and fresh basil.

LOW-SODIUM DINNER RECIPES

Baked Lemon Herb Chicken:

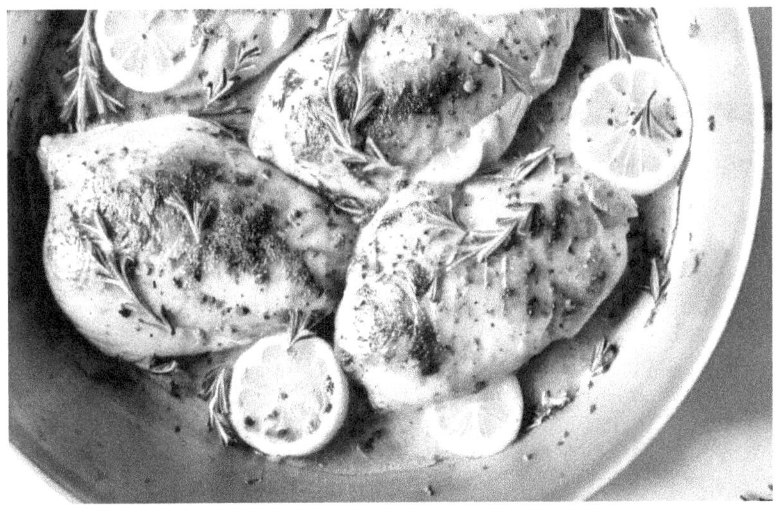

Ingredients: Chicken breasts, lemon, herbs (rosemary, thyme), olive oil.

Preparation: Marinate chicken with lemon, herbs, and olive oil; bake until cooked through.

Vegetarian Chickpea Stir-Fry:

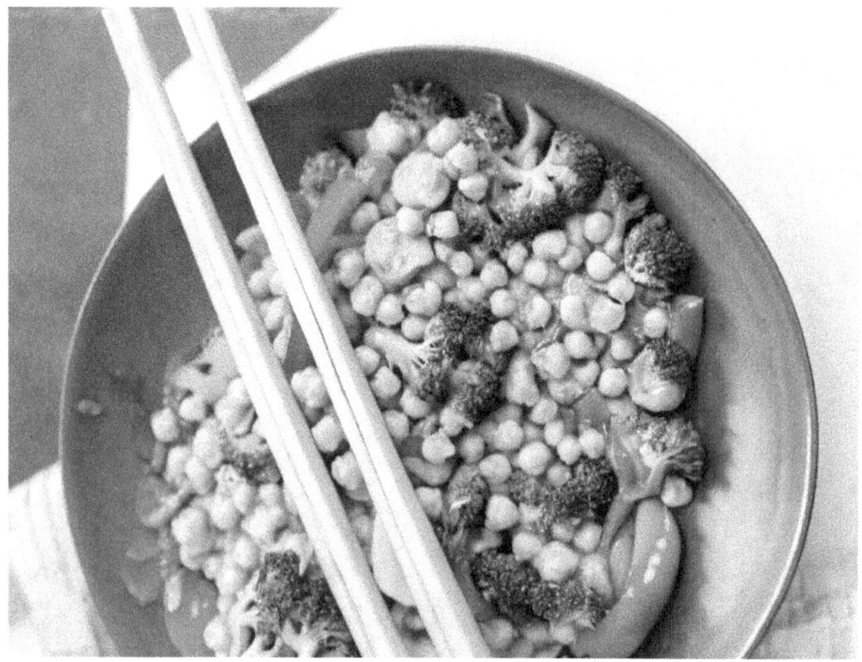

Ingredients: Chickpeas, broccoli, bell peppers, soy sauce.

Preparation: Stir-fry chickpeas with broccoli and bell peppers in soy sauce.

Salmon with Dill Sauce:

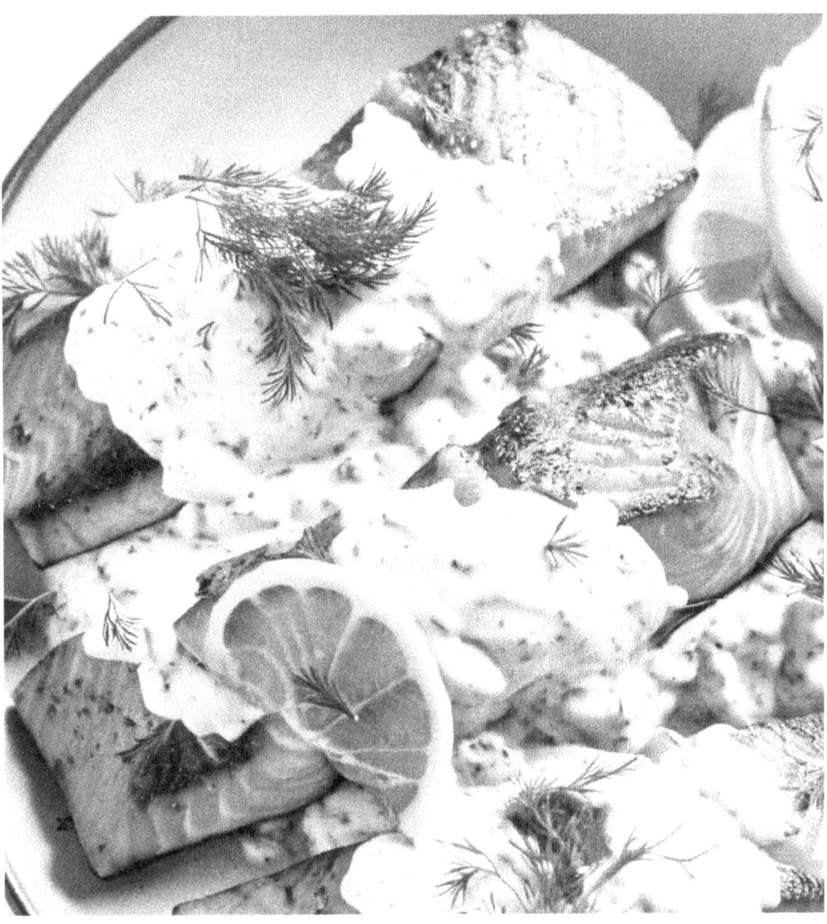

Ingredients: Salmon fillet, dill, Greek yogurt, lemon.

Preparation: Grill or bake salmon, top with a sauce made from dill, Greek yogurt, and lemon.

Eggplant and Tomato Stew:

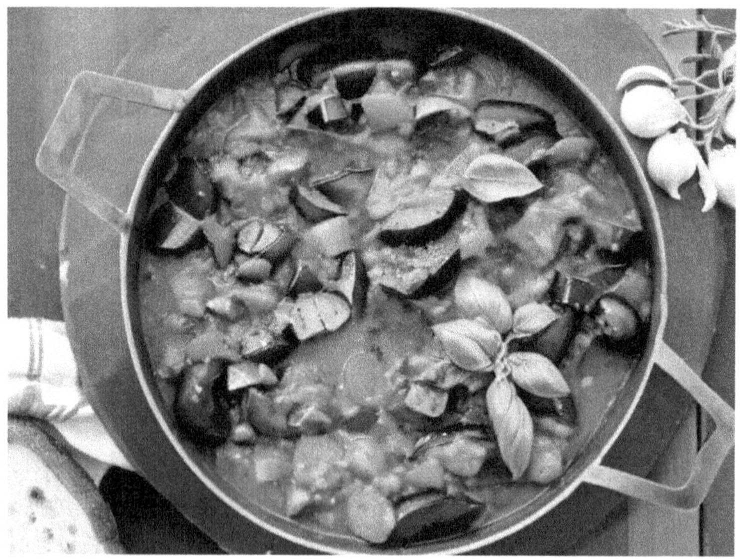

Ingredients: Eggplant, tomatoes, garlic, olive oil.

Preparation: Cook eggplant and tomatoes with minced garlic in olive oil.

Turkey and Vegetable Skillet:

Ingredients: Ground turkey, zucchini, tomatoes, Italian seasoning.

Preparation: Brown ground turkey, sauté with zucchini, tomatoes, and Italian seasoning.

Spaghetti Squash Primavera:

Ingredients: Spaghetti squash, cherry tomatoes, spinach, garlic.

Preparation: Roast spaghetti squash, sauté with cherry tomatoes, spinach, and minced garlic.

Cauliflower Rice Stir-Fry:

Ingredients: Cauliflower rice, mixed vegetables, low sodium soy sauce.

Preparation: Stir-fry cauliflower rice with mixed vegetables in low sodium soy sauce.

Lemon Garlic Shrimp Skewers:

Ingredients: Shrimp, lemon, garlic, olive oil.

Preparation: Marinate shrimp in a mixture of lemon, minced garlic, and olive oil; grill on skewers.

Chickpea and Spinach Curry:

Ingredients: Chickpeas, spinach, coconut milk, curry spices.

Preparation: Cook chickpeas and spinach in coconut milk with your favorite curry spices.

Baked Cod with Herbs:

Ingredients: Cod fillet, herbs (parsley, dill), lemon.

Preparation: Coat cod with chopped herbs and lemon, bake until flaky.

Vegetable and Tofu Kebabs:

Ingredients: Tofu, bell peppers, red onion, balsamic glaze.

Preparation: Skewer tofu, bell peppers, and red onion; grill and drizzle with balsamic glaze.

Lentil and Vegetable Soup:

Ingredients: Lentils, carrots, celery, low sodium vegetable broth.

Preparation: Cook lentils with diced carrots and celery in low sodium vegetable broth.

Stuffed Acorn Squash:

Ingredients: Acorn squash, quinoa, cranberries, walnuts.

Preparation: Roast acorn squash, fill with a mixture of cooked quinoa, cranberries, and chopped walnuts.

Balsamic Glazed Chicken Thighs:

Ingredients: Chicken thighs, balsamic vinegar, honey, garlic.

Preparation: Marinate chicken thighs in balsamic vinegar, honey, and minced garlic; bake until caramelized.

Mushroom and Spinach Risotto:

Ingredients: Arborio rice, mushrooms, spinach, vegetable broth.

Preparation: Sauté mushrooms and spinach, stir in cooked Arborio rice and vegetable broth.

Greek Lentil Salad:

Ingredients: Lentils, cucumbers, cherry tomatoes, feta cheese.

Preparation: Combine cooked lentils with diced cucumbers, cherry tomatoes, and crumbled feta.

Grilled Portobello Mushrooms:

Ingredients: Portobello mushrooms, balsamic vinegar, garlic.

Preparation: Grill portobello mushrooms marinated in balsamic vinegar and minced garlic.

Asian-Inspired Tofu Stir-Fry:

Ingredients: Tofu, broccoli, snap peas, low sodium soy sauce.

Preparation: Stir-fry tofu, broccoli, and snap peas in low sodium soy sauce.

Turkey and Sweet Potato Hash:

Ingredients: Ground turkey, sweet potatoes, bell peppers, cumin.

Preparation: Sauté ground turkey with diced sweet potatoes, bell peppers, and cumin.

Cabbage and Carrot Rolls with Turkey:

Ingredients: Cabbage leaves, ground turkey, carrots, tomato sauce.

Preparation: Fill cabbage leaves with a mixture of ground turkey, shredded carrots, and tomato sauce; bake until tender.

Lemon Herb Grilled Swordfish:

Ingredients: Swordfish steaks, lemon, herbs (thyme, rosemary).

Preparation: Marinate swordfish in lemon and chopped herbs; grill until cooked through.

Butternut Squash and Kale Risotto:

Ingredients: Arborio rice, butternut squash, kale, vegetable broth.

Preparation: Sauté butternut squash and kale, stir in cooked Arborio rice and vegetable broth.

Chili Lime Grilled Chicken:

Ingredients: Chicken breasts, chili powder, lime, olive oil.

Preparation: Marinate chicken in a mixture of chili powder, lime juice, and olive oil; grill until done.

Stuffed Zucchini Boats:

Ingredients: Zucchini, ground chicken, tomatoes, basil.

Preparation: Hollow out zucchini, fill with a mixture of cooked ground chicken, diced tomatoes, and chopped basil; bake until tender.

Mushroom and Spinach Quiche:

Ingredients: Whole wheat pie crust, eggs, mushrooms, spinach.

Preparation: Whisk eggs, mix with sautéed mushrooms and spinach, pour into pie crust, and bake.

Chickpea and Vegetable Curry:

Ingredients: Chickpeas, mixed vegetables, coconut milk, curry spices.

Preparation: Cook chickpeas and mixed vegetables in coconut milk with your favorite curry spices.

Honey Mustard Glazed Salmon:

Ingredients: Salmon fillet, honey, Dijon mustard, garlic.

Preparation: Mix honey, Dijon mustard, and minced garlic; brush over salmon and bake.

Vegetable and Brown Rice Casserole:

Ingredients: Brown rice, mixed vegetables, low sodium cheese.

Preparation: Mix cooked brown rice with mixed vegetables, top with low sodium cheese, and bake until melted.

A 7-DAY LOW SODIUM MEAL PLAN

Day	Breakfast	Lunch	Dinner
1	Oatmeal with Fresh Berries	Grilled Chicken Salad	Baked Lemon Herb Chicken
2	Greek Yogurt Parfait	Quinoa and Black Bean Bowl	Vegetarian Chickpea Stir-Fry
3	Avocado Toast	Salmon and Asparagus Foil Pack	Eggplant and Tomato Stew
4	Egg White Omelette	Vegetarian Wrap	Quinoa and Black Bean Stuffed Peppers
5	Smoothie Bowl	Mediterranean Chickpea Salad	Turkey and Vegetable Skillet
6	Quinoa Breakfast Bowl	Turkey and Avocado Lettuce Wraps	Spaghetti Squash Primavera
7	Chia Seed Pudding	Brown Rice and Vegetable Stir-Fry	Cauliflower Rice Stir-Fry

SIMPLE STRATEGIES TO CUT
YOUR SODIUM INTAKE

High sodium levels in the diet are often linked to hypertension, heart disease, and other health issues. Fortunately, implementing simple strategies to cut sodium intake doesn't mean sacrificing flavor or enjoyment in your meals. Here are some effective and straightforward approaches to reduce your sodium consumption and embark on a path to a healthier lifestyle.

1. Read Labels Mindfully: One of the simplest and most impactful strategies is to pay close attention to food labels. Many processed and packaged foods contain hidden sodium. Familiarize yourself with the terminology – sodium, sodium chloride, monosodium glutamate (MSG), and baking soda are all indicators of sodium content. Opt for products labeled as "low-sodium" or "sodium-free" whenever possible.

2. Cook at Home: Controlling your sodium intake becomes significantly easier when you prepare meals at home. Cooking from scratch allows you to choose fresh, whole ingredients and gives you full control over the amount of salt added to your dishes. Experiment with herbs, spices, citrus, and other flavor enhancers to make your meals delicious without relying on excessive sodium.

3. Use Herbs and Spices Creatively: Herbs and spices are your allies in the quest for flavorful, low-sodium meals. From basil and thyme to cumin and paprika, the world of herbs and spices is vast and diverse. Experiment with different combinations to discover new and exciting flavor profiles. Fresh herbs, in particular, can add vibrancy to your dishes while minimizing the need for added salt.

4. Gradual Reduction of Salt: If you're accustomed to heavily salted meals, consider gradually reducing the amount of salt you use. This allows your taste buds to adjust to lower sodium levels over time. You might find that you need less salt than you initially thought to enjoy the natural flavors of food.

5. Be Wary of Condiments and Sauces: Many condiments and sauces, such as soy sauce, ketchup, and salad dressings, are significant sources of hidden sodium. Opt for low-sodium or sodium-free versions, or try making your own sauces at home using fresh ingredients. Experimenting with homemade dressings and marinades gives you control over the sodium content while adding a personalized touch to your meals.

6. Choose Fresh Produce: Incorporating a variety of fresh fruits and vegetables into your diet not only provides essential nutrients but also helps naturally lower sodium intake. Fresh produce is naturally low in sodium and high in potassium, which has been associated with lower blood pressure.

7. Rethink Canned and Processed Foods: Canned and processed foods often contain high levels of sodium for preservation and flavor enhancement. Whenever possible, choose fresh or frozen alternatives. If you need to use canned items, rinse them under water to remove excess salt before incorporating them into your recipes.

8. Mindful Dining Out: When dining out, ask for your dish to be prepared with minimal or no added salt. Choose restaurants that offer healthier and lower-sodium options. Additionally, consider sharing large portions or taking half of your meal home to manage your sodium intake effectively.

9. Stay Hydrated: Drinking an adequate amount of water helps flush excess sodium from your body. Staying hydrated is an essential component of any low-sodium lifestyle. Opt for water instead of sugary or high-sodium beverages to maintain proper fluid balance.

10. Educate Yourself: Lastly, continue educating yourself on the sodium content of various foods and how it can impact your health. Being informed allows you to make conscious choices about your diet and empowers you to prioritize long-term well-being.

Flavor Enhancers That Go Beyond Salt:

1. **Citrus Zest:** The zest of citrus fruits such as lemons, limes, and oranges can add a burst of flavor to dishes. Grate the outer peel to infuse your meals with a refreshing and zesty essence.

2. **Vinegar Varieties:** Different types of vinegar, including balsamic, apple cider, and rice vinegar, offer unique flavors that enhance your dishes. Use them in dressings, marinades, and sauces for a tangy kick.

3. **Garlic and Onions:** Fresh garlic and onions are aromatic additions that contribute rich flavors to savory dishes. Sauté them to build a strong foundation for soups, stews, and sauces.

4. **Herb Infused Oils:** Infuse olive oil with herbs like basil, thyme, or rosemary to create herb-infused oils. Drizzle these oils over salads, vegetables, or grilled proteins for an elevated taste.

5. **Mustard:** Dijon, whole grain, or spicy mustard can serve as excellent alternatives to traditional sodium-laden condiments. Mustard brings a robust and pungent flavor that complements various dishes.

6. **Cumin and Smoked Paprika:** These spices add a smoky and earthy depth to your meals. Sprinkle cumin and smoked paprika on roasted vegetables, meats, or grains to impart a distinctive flavor.

7. **Fresh Ginger:** Grated or minced fresh ginger brings a warm and slightly spicy element to both savory and sweet dishes. It pairs well with Asian-inspired recipes and can be used in teas, stir-fries, and marinades.

Cutting sodium intake doesn't have to be a daunting task. By adopting these simple strategies, you can create a sustainable and enjoyable low-sodium lifestyle that contributes to better health and vitality. Making informed choices about your food, experimenting with flavors, and gradually reducing salt will not only benefit your heart but also enhance your appreciation for the rich and diverse world of culinary delights.

The Quick Fix Low Sodium Cookbook

DISPELLING MYTHS AROUND SALT CONSUMPTION

Misconception 1: All Sodium is Harmful

Fact: Not all sodium is created equal. Sodium is an essential electrolyte that plays a vital role in maintaining fluid balance, nerve function, and muscle contractions. However, the source of sodium matters. Natural sources like fruits, vegetables, and unprocessed meats contain sodium in amounts that support bodily functions without leading to excessive intake. The real concern lies in the overconsumption of sodium from processed and packaged foods, where salt is often used as a preservative and flavor enhancer.

Misconception 2: Sea Salt is Healthier than Table Salt

Fact: Sea salt and table salt are nutritionally similar. While sea salt is often perceived as a healthier alternative to table salt, both contain comparable amounts of sodium by weight. Sea salt may have trace minerals that add a subtle flavor, but the nutritional difference between the two is minimal. Regardless of the type of salt you choose, moderation is key.

Misconception 3: Cutting Out Salt Means Sacrificing Flavor

Fact: Flavor can be enhanced without excessive salt. Many people believe that reducing sodium in their diet equates to bland and tasteless meals. However, there are numerous flavor enhancers beyond salt that can elevate your culinary experience. Herbs, spices, citrus, garlic, and vinegar can add depth and complexity to dishes without relying on excessive sodium. Experimenting with these alternatives allows you to discover new and exciting flavors.

Misconception 4: Low-Sodium Diets are Only for Those with High Blood Pressure

Fact: Low-sodium diets benefit everyone. While it's true that reducing sodium intake is particularly crucial for individuals with hypertension or heart conditions, everyone can benefit from a mindful approach to sodium consumption. Excessive sodium intake is associated with various health issues, including kidney problems and an increased risk of stroke. Adopting a low-sodium diet promotes overall well-being and reduces the risk of developing these health concerns.

Misconception 5: Processed Foods Without a Salty Taste Are Low in Sodium

Fact: Processed foods can be high in hidden sodium. The taste of salt is not always an accurate indicator of sodium content. Many processed foods, even those that don't taste particularly salty, can be loaded with hidden sodium. This includes items like canned soups, sauces, and ready-made meals. Checking nutrition labels for sodium content is crucial to making informed choices.

Misconception 6: Athletes Need High-Sodium Diets

Fact: Athletes can meet sodium needs without excessive intake. While athletes may lose sodium through sweat during intense workouts, it doesn't mean they need excessively high-sodium diets. Balanced nutrition that includes sodium from natural sources like fruits, vegetables, and whole grains can adequately meet their needs. Excessive sodium intake can lead to dehydration and negatively impact overall health.

Misconception 7: Salt Substitutes are Always a Healthy Option

Fact: Salt substitutes may contain potassium. Some salt substitutes replace sodium with potassium, which can be a healthier alternative for certain individuals, especially those with high blood pressure. However, individuals with kidney problems or those taking medications that affect potassium levels should consult with a healthcare professional before using salt substitutes. It's essential to choose substitutes carefully and be aware of their potential impact on overall health.

Separating Fact from Fiction:

1. **Understanding Optimal Sodium Intake:** The American Heart Association recommends a daily sodium intake of no more than 2,300 milligrams, with an ideal target of 1,500 milligrams for most adults. This guideline emphasizes the importance of moderation rather than complete elimination.

2. **Differentiating Between Natural and Added Sodium:** Natural sodium, found in whole foods like fruits, vegetables, and dairy, is accompanied by essential

nutrients. It's the added or processed sodium that can lead to health concerns. Reading labels helps identify hidden sources of added sodium in various food products.

3. **Balancing Sodium with Other Minerals:** Sodium works in tandem with other minerals like potassium. Balancing sodium intake with an increased consumption of potassium-rich foods, such as bananas, leafy greens, and sweet potatoes, is crucial for overall health.

4. **Mindful Consumption of Processed Foods:** While it's advisable to minimize processed foods, not all of them are sodium-laden. Opting for lower-sodium versions and being aware of serving sizes can help incorporate some processed foods into a balanced diet without excessive sodium intake.

5. **Gradual Reduction is Sustainable:** Rather than drastic and unsustainable changes, gradually reducing sodium intake is a more practical approach. This allows taste buds to adjust, making long-term adherence to a lower-sodium lifestyle more feasible.

CONCLUSION

A heart-healthy lifestyle is built on conscious choices, and one pivotal aspect is the reduction of sodium intake. The journey towards easy, delicious, and heart-healthy eating begins with simple strategies that not only benefit cardiovascular health but also enhance the overall well-being of individuals. Here's a guide to navigating this journey, making mindful choices, and savoring the flavors of a heart-healthy lifestyle.

1. Start with Conscious Choices: The first step towards a heart-healthy lifestyle is making conscious choices. Understanding the impact of sodium on heart health empowers individuals to take control of their dietary habits. By opting for low-sodium alternatives and being mindful of hidden sodium sources, individuals can lay the foundation for a heart-conscious approach to eating.

2. Whole Foods as the Cornerstone: Whole, unprocessed foods form the cornerstone of a heart-healthy diet. Fruits, vegetables, whole grains, lean proteins, and nuts provide essential nutrients without the excessive sodium often found in processed foods. These foods are not only nutritious but also delicious, offering a vibrant array of flavors that can be appreciated without relying on added salt.

3. Culinary Creativity with Fresh Herbs and Spices: Herbs and spices become invaluable allies in the quest for reducing sodium without sacrificing taste. The culinary world is rich with options – basil, cilantro, thyme, rosemary, cumin, and turmeric are just a few examples. Experimenting with these flavor enhancers opens up a palette of possibilities, allowing individuals to create exciting, satisfying meals that tickle the taste buds.

4. Balanced Nutritional Choices: Achieving a heart-healthy lifestyle involves not just reducing sodium but also maintaining a well-balanced diet. Nutrient-dense foods, rich in vitamins, minerals, and antioxidants, contribute to overall cardiovascular health.

Balancing macronutrients – proteins, carbohydrates, and fats – supports a holistic approach to well-being.

5. Practical Tips for Low-Sodium Cooking: Practical tips make low-sodium cooking accessible and enjoyable. Rinsing canned goods, choosing fresh over processed, and reading labels attentively are fundamental practices. Gradually reducing salt usage in recipes allows the palate to adapt to lower sodium levels without compromising on flavor.

6. The Pleasure of Home Cooking: The heart-healthy journey thrives in the heart of the home – the kitchen. Cooking at home not only provides control over ingredients but also fosters a deeper connection with the food being consumed. Embracing the joy of home-cooked meals encourages individuals to appreciate the nourishment derived from fresh, wholesome ingredients.

7. Mindful Dining Out: While home-cooked meals are a cornerstone, dining out is an inevitable part of modern living. Choosing restaurants that prioritize heart-healthy options, asking for meals to be prepared with minimal salt, and being aware of portion sizes contribute to a mindful dining-out experience.

8. Hydration Habits: Hydration plays a crucial role in a heart-healthy lifestyle. Opting for water over sugary or sodium-laden beverages ensures proper fluid balance. Staying well-hydrated supports overall health and complements dietary efforts aimed at reducing sodium intake.

9. Community Support and Education: Embarking on a heart-healthy journey is often more successful when supported by a community. Sharing experiences, recipes, and tips with like-minded individuals fosters motivation and a sense of collective achievement. Staying informed through ongoing education ensures that individuals remain empowered to make informed choices about their heart health.

10. Celebrate Progress, Not Perfection: Finally, embracing a heart-healthy lifestyle is a journey, not a destination. Celebrate progress, no matter how small, and recognize that each step towards mindful eating contributes to overall well-being. Cultivating a positive relationship with food and appreciating the journey makes the pursuit of a heart-healthy lifestyle a fulfilling and sustainable endeavor.

Thanking You

The Quick Fix Low Sodium Cookbook

As you embark on your journey toward easy, delicious, and heart-healthy eating, we extend our heartfelt gratitude for choosing our guide to cut sodium intake. Your commitment to prioritizing your health is commendable, and we are here to support you every step of the way.

Wishing you success on your path to a heart-healthy lifestyle! We trust that the strategies and recipes provided will not only make a positive impact on your sodium intake but also bring joy to your culinary experiences. Our goal is to empower you with the knowledge and tools to make informed choices that contribute to your overall well-being.

If you find value in "The Quick Fix Low Sodium Cookbook" and the strategies shared within, **we invite you to leave a comment or review.** *Your feedback is invaluable, not only for us but for others on a similar journey.*

Share your experiences, the recipes you loved, and any insights gained during your exploration of heart-healthy eating.

Once again, thank you for entrusting us with a part of your health journey. Here's to your success, well-being, and the delicious discoveries that lie ahead!